CONTENTS

INTRODUCTION

Welcome to "The Interstitial Cystitis Diet: Nourishing Solutions for Managing Symptoms." If you are reading this book, chances are you or someone you care about is dealing with the challenges of interstitial cystitis (IC). Living with IC can be a journey filled with discomfort, pain, and frustration, but there is hope. By understanding the role of diet in managing IC symptoms, you can take an active role in improving your quality of life.

This book is designed to be your comprehensive guide to the interstitial cystitis diet—an approach that focuses on identifying and avoiding foods and beverages that may trigger or worsen IC symptoms while incorporating nourishing and supportive options. It aims to provide you with the knowledge, tools, and practical strategies to make informed dietary choices that can positively impact your IC symptoms.

Throughout the pages of this book, we will explore the connection between IC and diet, shedding light on the foods that can either aggravate or soothe IC symptoms. We will delve into the underlying mechanisms of IC, understanding the role of inflammation and potential triggers that can exacerbate urinary discomfort and pain.

You will learn about common food irritants and triggers that IC patients often face, enabling you to navigate your grocery store aisles with confidence and make choices that are kind to your bladder. We will discuss the impact of various food groups on IC symptoms, providing you with a comprehensive understanding of how different foods can affect your well-being.

But this book is not just about restrictions and limitations. We will also highlight a wide range of IC-friendly foods that you can enjoy, ensuring you receive the necessary nutrients while minimizing symptom triggers. From delicious recipes to meal planning tips, we will help you create a balanced and satisfying diet that supports your overall health and well-being.

Furthermore, we recognize that each person's experience with IC is unique, and what works for one may not work for another. That's why we encourage you to work closely with healthcare professionals and registered dietitians who specialize in IC to tailor the dietary approach to your specific needs.

Living with IC can be challenging, but by embracing an IC-friendly diet, you are taking a significant step toward managing your symptoms and regaining control over your life. We hope that this book serves as a source of knowledge, inspiration, and empowerment as you embark on your journey to find relief and live a fulfilling life with IC.

Remember, you are not alone in this. Together, we can navigate the complexities of the interstitial cystitis diet and discover nourishing solutions that help you thrive. Let's embark on this transformative journey towards a healthier, more vibrant life with interstitial cystitis.

CHAPTER ONE

Introduction

Explanation of interstitial cystitis

(IC) and its impact on daily life

Interstitial cystitis (IC), also known as painful bladder syndrome, is a chronic condition that affects the bladder, causing pain, discomfort, and frequent urination. It is a complex condition with no known exact cause, but it is believed to involve a combination of factors, including bladder inflammation and dysfunction. IC predominantly affects women, although men can also develop the condition.

The symptoms of IC can vary from person to person, and the severity can range from mild discomfort to debilitating pain. Common symptoms include pelvic pain, urinary urgency and frequency, and pain or discomfort during sexual intercourse. These symptoms can significantly impact a person's daily life, affecting their physical, emotional, and social well-being.

Living with IC can be challenging due to the chronic pain and discomfort it causes. Individuals with IC often experience sleep disturbances and fatigue, making it difficult to engage in daily activities. The need for frequent bathroom breaks to relieve urinary urgency can disrupt work, school, and social engagements. The unpredictability of IC flares can lead to increased stress and anxiety, as individuals never know when their symptoms may worsen.

IC can also interfere with intimacy and sexual relationships. The pain and discomfort experienced during sexual intercourse can make it difficult to engage in or enjoy sexual activities. This aspect of IC can strain relationships and lead to feelings of frustration and isolation.

The emotional toll of living with IC should not be underestimated. The chronic nature of the condition can lead to feelings of helplessness, frustration, and depression. The financial burden of managing IC can also be significant, with costs associated with doctor visits, medications, treatments, and necessary lifestyle adjustments.

Furthermore, IC can have an impact on relationships with family and friends. Individuals with IC may need to limit their activities or cancel plans due to symptom flares, which can lead to feelings of guilt and isolation. This can strain relationships and make it challenging to maintain a social life.

In addition to the physical and emotional impact, IC can also affect one's ability to travel or participate in recreational activities. The fear of symptom flares or the need for constant access to restrooms can limit opportunities for enjoyment and exploration. This can further contribute to feelings of isolation and a decreased quality of life.

Managing IC requires a multidimensional approach. While there is currently no cure for IC, various treatment options are available to help manage symptoms and improve quality of life. These can include dietary modifications, physical therapy, medication, bladder instillations, nerve stimulation, and in severe cases, surgery. However, finding the most effective treatment or combination of treatments may take time and require ongoing adjustments.

Self-care strategies are also important in managing IC symptoms. Stress management techniques, relaxation exercises, and maintaining a healthy lifestyle can all play a significant role in symptom management and overall well-being. It is crucial for individuals with IC to establish a network of healthcare professionals who specialize in the condition to ensure proper management and support.

Education and awareness about IC are essential in promoting understanding and empathy for those living with the condition. The IC community, including support groups and online forums, can provide valuable resources, information, and a sense of belonging for individuals seeking support.

While living with IC can be challenging, many individuals are able to find relief and lead fulfilling lives through proper management and support. Ongoing research into the causes and treatment of IC offers hope for improved therapies and potential future breakthroughs. It is important for individuals with IC to advocate for themselves, communicate their needs to healthcare providers, and actively participate in their treatment plans.

In conclusion, interstitial cystitis (IC) is a chronic condition that affects the bladder, causing pain, discomfort, and frequent urination. It can have a significant impact on daily life, affecting physical well-being, emotional health, and social relationships. However, with proper management, support, and self-care strategies, individuals with IC can find relief and improve their quality of life. While there is no cure for IC, various treatment options are available to manage symptoms and minimize their impact on daily life.

One of the key aspects of managing IC is developing a comprehensive treatment plan in collaboration with healthcare professionals. This plan may include dietary modifications, as certain foods and beverages can trigger IC symptoms. Common triggers include acidic foods, caffeine, artificial sweeteners, spicy foods, and alcohol. By identifying and avoiding these triggers, individuals with IC can reduce symptom flare-ups and improve their overall well-being.

In addition to dietary changes, physical therapy can be beneficial for IC patients. Pelvic floor physical therapy focuses on strengthening and relaxing the muscles in the pelvic region, which can help alleviate pain and improve bladder function. Physical therapists can provide guidance on specific exercises and techniques tailored to the individual's needs.

Medications may also be prescribed to manage IC symptoms. These can include oral medications to reduce inflammation, relieve pain, and control bladder spasms. In some cases, medications may be administered directly into the bladder through instillations to provide localized relief. It is important to work closely with a healthcare provider to determine the most suitable medication options and dosages.

For individuals with severe and refractory IC, more invasive treatments such as nerve stimulation or surgery may be considered. Nerve stimulation involves the implantation of a device that delivers electrical impulses to the nerves controlling the bladder, helping to alleviate symptoms. Surgical interventions are generally considered when other treatments have not been successful and may involve bladder augmentation or removal in extreme cases.

Living with IC also requires proactive self-care strategies. Managing stress levels is crucial, as stress can exacerbate symptoms. Engaging in stress reduction techniques such as meditation, deep breathing exercises, and mindfulness can help individuals cope with the emotional and physical challenges associated with IC.

Support from family, friends, and support groups can make a significant difference in an individual's ability to cope with IC. Sharing experiences, learning from others, and receiving emotional support can help individuals feel less isolated and better equipped to manage the impact of IC on their daily lives.

Education is key in empowering individuals with IC to take control of their condition. Understanding the nature of IC, its triggers, and treatment options enables individuals to make informed decisions and actively participate in their care. Staying updated on the latest research and developments in IC treatment can also provide hope for new therapies or approaches on the horizon.

While living with IC can be challenging, it is important to remain optimistic and maintain a positive mindset. Every individual's journey with IC is unique, and what works for one person may not work for another. Patience, perseverance, and self-compassion are crucial when navigating the complexities of managing IC.

In conclusion, interstitial cystitis (IC) is a chronic condition that significantly impacts daily life. Its symptoms can cause pain, discomfort, and disruptions in various aspects of life, including physical, emotional, and social well-being. However, with a multidimensional approach that includes treatment options, self-care strategies, and a support network, individuals with IC can find relief, improve their quality of life, and regain a sense of control over their condition. By actively managing IC and staying informed about advancements in treatment, individuals can lead fulfilling lives despite the challenges posed by this chronic condition.

Importance of diet in managing IC symptoms

The importance of diet in managing interstitial cystitis (IC) symptoms cannot be overstated. Diet plays a crucial role in alleviating symptoms, reducing inflammation, and improving the overall well-being of individuals with IC. Understanding and implementing an IC-friendly diet can make a significant difference in managing the condition effectively. Here are some key reasons why diet is essential in managing IC symptoms:

- Reducing Irritation: Certain foods and beverages can irritate the bladder, leading to increased inflammation and worsening of IC symptoms. By identifying and avoiding these trigger foods, individuals can minimize bladder irritation and reduce symptom flare-ups. Common trigger foods include acidic foods (such as citrus fruits and tomatoes), spicy foods, caffeine, alcohol, carbonated beverages, artificial sweeteners, and certain preservatives.

- Decreasing Inflammation: Inflammation is a key factor in IC, and certain foods have the potential to either promote or reduce inflammation in the body. An anti-inflammatory diet can help reduce overall inflammation levels, leading to a decrease in IC symptoms. Foods rich in antioxidants, such as fruits and vegetables, whole grains, lean proteins, and healthy fats (like omega-3 fatty acids), can help reduce inflammation and promote healing.

- Balancing pH Levels: The pH level of urine can have an impact on IC symptoms. Consuming alkaline foods can help balance the pH levels in the urine, reducing bladder irritation and discomfort. Alkaline foods include leafy greens, cucumbers, celery, watermelon, and certain nuts and seeds. On the other hand, acidic foods like citrus fruits, cranberries, and vinegar can increase the acidity of urine and potentially worsen IC symptoms.

- Identifying Personal Triggers: Each individual

with IC may have specific food triggers that exacerbate their symptoms. Keeping a food diary and tracking symptoms can help identify personal triggers. By noting the foods consumed and the subsequent symptom flare-ups, individuals can pinpoint their specific triggers and make informed dietary adjustments.

- Supporting Gut Health: The gut and the bladder are closely interconnected, and an unhealthy gut can contribute to inflammation and worsen IC symptoms. A diet that supports gut health, including the consumption of fiber-rich foods, probiotics, and fermented foods, can promote a healthy balance of gut bacteria, enhance digestion, and potentially reduce IC symptoms.

- Nutritional Support: Following an IC-friendly diet does not mean compromising on nutrition. It is important to ensure that the diet includes a variety of nutrient-dense foods to meet the body's nutritional needs. This can be achieved by incorporating a wide range of fruits, vegetables, lean proteins, whole grains, and healthy fats. Nutritional deficiencies can impact overall health and potentially exacerbate IC symptoms.

- Individualized Approach: While there are general guidelines for an IC-friendly diet, it is important to recognize that each individual's tolerance for specific foods may vary. Some individuals may find relief by eliminating certain trigger foods, while others may need to experiment further and identify additional personalized triggers. Working with a healthcare professional, such as a registered dietitian or nutritionist, can help tailor an IC diet to meet individual needs.

- Empowerment and Control: Adhering to an IC-friendly diet gives individuals a sense of empowerment and control over their condition. By making conscious choices about what they eat, individuals can actively manage their symptoms and potentially reduce the frequency and intensity of IC flares. It provides individuals with a proactive role in their own well-being and instills a sense of hope and optimism.

It is important to note that dietary changes alone may not be sufficient to manage IC symptoms for everyone. Treatment plans may also include other interventions, such as medication, physical therapy, stress management techniques, and lifestyle modifications. However, diet serves as a foundational component and complements other treatment strategies in achieving optimal symptom management and overall well-being.

When embarking on an IC-friendly diet, it is essential to approach it with patience and an open mind. It may take time to identify personal triggers and determine the foods that work best for individual symptom management. Keeping a food diary and working closely with a healthcare professional can provide valuable guidance and support throughout the process.

In addition to avoiding trigger foods, there are various dietary strategies that can be beneficial for individuals with IC:

- Hydration: Maintaining adequate hydration is crucial for bladder health. Drinking plenty of water throughout the day can help dilute urine and reduce bladder irritation. However, it is important to avoid excessive fluid intake that may increase urinary frequency and urgency.
- Balanced Meals: Building meals that include a combination of lean proteins, whole grains, healthy fats, and a variety of fruits and vegetables can provide essential nutrients while minimizing potential triggers. This balanced approach ensures a wide range of vitamins, minerals, and antioxidants necessary for overall health.
- Cooking Methods: Choosing appropriate cooking methods can help minimize irritation. Steaming, baking, grilling, or boiling foods are generally better options than frying or sautéing, as they reduce the formation of potentially irritating compounds.
- Alternative Ingredients: Exploring alternative ingredients can open up a world of possibilities for delicious and IC-friendly meals. For example, substituting citrus fruits with non-acidic alternatives like pears or using herbs and spices to add flavor instead of spicy seasonings can help reduce symptom triggers.

- Mindful Eating: Practicing mindful eating techniques can promote better digestion and help individuals listen to their body's signals. Eating slowly, chewing thoroughly, and paying attention to portion sizes can aid in better digestion and reduce potential discomfort.
- Individualized Approach: It is important to recognize that each person with IC may have unique dietary tolerances and triggers. What works for one individual may not work for another. Therefore, an individualized approach that takes into account personal experiences and symptoms is crucial.

It is worth noting that dietary modifications alone may not completely eliminate IC symptoms. The goal is to minimize triggers, reduce inflammation, and support overall well-being. It is often a combination of various treatment strategies, including medications, lifestyle modifications, and stress management techniques, that lead to optimal symptom management.

In conclusion, diet plays a vital role in managing IC symptoms and improving the overall quality of life for individuals with the condition. By identifying trigger foods, reducing inflammation, supporting gut health, and adopting a balanced and individualized approach, individuals can significantly alleviate symptoms and take an active role in their own well-being. While dietary modifications are an essential component, they work synergistically with other treatment strategies to provide comprehensive symptom management for interstitial cystitis. Consulting with healthcare professionals and seeking guidance from registered dietitians or nutritionists can provide personalized support on the journey towards optimal IC symptom management through dietary modifications.

Understanding Interstitial Cystitis

Overview of interstitial cystitis: causes, symptoms, and diagnosis

Interstitial cystitis (IC), also known as painful bladder syndrome, is a chronic condition that affects the bladder and causes pain, discomfort, and urinary symptoms. It is a complex and poorly understood condition with no definitive cause, but it is believed to involve a combination of factors including bladder inflammation, dysfunction of the protective lining of the bladder, and underlying changes in the nerves and muscles of the bladder.

Causes of Interstitial Cystitis:

The exact cause of IC remains unknown, but several theories have been proposed. Potential causes and contributing factors include:

- Bladder Lining Defects: It is suggested that defects in the protective lining of the bladder, known as the urothelium, may allow toxic substances in urine to irritate the bladder wall and cause inflammation.
- Autoimmune Reaction: Some researchers speculate that IC may be an autoimmune condition, where the immune system mistakenly attacks the bladder tissues, leading to inflammation and pain.
- Nerve Abnormalities: Nerve-related abnormalities, such as increased nerve growth or altered signaling between the bladder and brain, may play a role in IC development and symptom generation.
- Pelvic Floor Dysfunction: Dysfunction of the pelvic floor muscles, which support the bladder and other pelvic organs, may contribute to IC symptoms.
- Genetic Predisposition: There is evidence to suggest that certain genetic factors may predispose individuals to developing IC, although further research is needed to fully understand these connections.

Symptoms of Interstitial Cystitis:

The symptoms of IC can vary in intensity and presentation

among individuals. They may also fluctuate over time, with periods of remission followed by symptom flare-ups. Common symptoms of IC include:

- Chronic Pelvic Pain: The hallmark symptom of IC is chronic pain in the pelvic region, including the bladder, lower abdomen, and perineal area. The pain can range from mild discomfort to severe and debilitating.
- Urgency and Frequency: Individuals with IC often experience a frequent need to urinate (urinary frequency), and a sense of urgency to urinate even with small volumes of urine in the bladder. This can significantly disrupt daily activities and sleep patterns.
- Painful Bladder Filling: Some individuals with IC experience pain or discomfort as the bladder fills with urine, leading to the need for frequent urination to relieve the discomfort.
- Painful Sexual Intercourse: IC can cause pain or discomfort during sexual intercourse, leading to decreased sexual desire and intimacy.
- Nocturia: Many individuals with IC wake up during the night to urinate (nocturia), which can further disrupt sleep patterns.
- Emotional and Psychological Impact: Living with chronic pain and disruptive urinary symptoms can lead to emotional distress, anxiety, and depression.

Diagnosis of Interstitial Cystitis:

Diagnosing IC can be challenging as there is no specific

test that can definitively confirm the condition. Diagnosis is typically based on a combination of medical history, symptom evaluation, and exclusion of other possible causes of symptoms. The diagnostic process may involve the following:

- Medical History and Symptom Assessment: A healthcare professional will review the patient's medical history, including symptoms, their frequency and duration, and the impact on daily life. Detailed information about urinary habits, pain patterns, and potential triggers will be obtained.
- Physical Examination: A physical examination may be performed to assess the pelvic area for any signs of tenderness, pain, or abnormalities.
- Urinalysis and Urine Culture: These tests are conducted to rule out urinary tract infections or other underlying conditions that may cause similar symptoms.
- Cystoscopy: This procedure involves the insertion of a thin, flexible tube with a camera (cystoscope) into the bladder through the urethra. Cystoscopy allows the healthcare professional to visually examine the bladder for signs of inflammation, ulcers, or other abnormalities associated with IC. In some cases, a hydrodistention may be performed during cystoscopy, where the bladder is filled with water to stretch and evaluate its capacity and response.
- Biopsy: A bladder biopsy may be performed

during cystoscopy to examine the bladder tissue under a microscope. This can help rule out other conditions and provide further evidence of inflammation or abnormalities associated with IC.

- Voiding Diary: Keeping a voiding diary, which involves recording the timing and volume of urine voided, can provide valuable information about urinary frequency, urgency, and patterns of symptom exacerbation.
- Potassium Sensitivity Test: This test involves the instillation of a solution containing potassium into the bladder, followed by assessment of any pain or discomfort experienced by the individual. Increased pain or urgency in response to the solution may suggest a diagnosis of IC.
- Pelvic Floor Evaluation: In some cases, an evaluation of the pelvic floor muscles may be conducted to assess for any abnormalities or dysfunction that may contribute to IC symptoms.

It is important to note that the diagnosis of IC is often one of exclusion, as there is no definitive test or biomarker for the condition. Healthcare professionals must rule out other possible causes of symptoms, such as urinary tract infections, bladder stones, or other bladder conditions that may present with similar symptoms.

In conclusion, interstitial cystitis (IC) is a chronic condition characterized by bladder inflammation and the presence of various urinary symptoms. While the exact cause remains unknown, it is believed to involve a combination of factors, including bladder lining defects, autoimmune reactions, nerve abnormalities, pelvic floor dysfunction, and genetic predisposition. The symptoms of IC can significantly impact an individual's quality of life, causing chronic pain, urinary urgency and frequency, discomfort during bladder filling, and disturbances in sexual function. Diagnosis of IC involves a comprehensive evaluation of medical history, symptom assessment, physical examination, urinalysis, cystoscopy, and potentially other tests to exclude other possible causes of symptoms. A multidisciplinary approach involving healthcare professionals, such as urologists, gynecologists, and pain specialists, is often necessary for proper diagnosis and management of IC. By understanding the causes, recognizing the symptoms, and undergoing a thorough diagnostic process, individuals with IC can receive appropriate treatment and support to manage their symptoms and improve their overall well-being.

The role of inflammation in IC

and its connection to diet

The role of inflammation in interstitial cystitis (IC) is significant and plays a crucial role in the development and progression of the condition. Inflammation refers to the body's response to injury or irritation, characterized by redness, swelling, pain, and heat. In the case of IC, chronic inflammation within the bladder wall contributes to the characteristic symptoms experienced by individuals with the condition.

The exact cause of the inflammation in IC is not fully understood, but it is believed to be multifactorial. One proposed theory is that defects in the protective lining of the bladder, called the urothelium, allow toxic substances in the urine to irritate the bladder wall and trigger an inflammatory response. This chronic inflammation can lead to further damage to the urothelium and perpetuate a cycle of inflammation and symptoms.

- Diet plays a critical role in managing IC symptoms by modulating inflammation levels in the body. Certain foods can either promote or reduce inflammation, and individuals with IC can benefit from an anti-inflammatory diet that helps minimize inflammation and alleviate symptoms. Here's how diet can impact inflammation in IC:

- Avoiding Trigger Foods: Certain foods are known to trigger inflammation in the bladder and worsen IC symptoms. These trigger foods can vary from person to person, but common culprits include acidic foods (such as citrus fruits, tomatoes, and vinegar), spicy foods, caffeine, alcohol, carbonated beverages, artificial sweeteners, and foods high in preservatives. By identifying and eliminating these trigger foods from the diet, individuals can reduce bladder irritation and lower inflammation levels.

- Anti-Inflammatory Foods: Incorporating anti-inflammatory foods into the diet can help counteract the inflammatory response in IC. These foods include fruits and vegetables rich in antioxidants, such as berries, leafy greens, and cruciferous vegetables. Healthy fats, like those found in fatty fish (salmon, mackerel, sardines), nuts, seeds, and olive oil, are also beneficial due to their omega-3 fatty acid content, which has anti-inflammatory properties. Whole grains and lean proteins can provide additional anti-inflammatory nutrients.

- Omega-3 Fatty Acids: Omega-3 fatty acids, found in fatty fish, flaxseeds, chia seeds, and walnuts, have been shown to have anti-inflammatory effects. These fatty acids help reduce the production of pro-inflammatory molecules in the body, thereby lowering inflammation levels. Including foods rich in omega-3 fatty acids in the diet can be beneficial for individuals with IC.

- Phytochemicals and Polyphenols: Many plant-based foods contain natural compounds known as phytochemicals and polyphenols, which have anti-inflammatory properties. Examples include turmeric, ginger, green tea, berries, and dark chocolate. These foods can help reduce inflammation and promote overall health.

- Hydration: Staying properly hydrated is crucial for managing IC symptoms and reducing inflammation. Drinking an adequate amount of water helps dilute urine, reducing bladder irritation and inflammation. It is important to note that hydration should be balanced, avoiding excessive fluid intake that may increase urinary frequency and urgency.

- Alkaline Diet: Some research suggests that maintaining a slightly alkaline pH level in urine may help reduce inflammation and IC symptoms. Consuming alkaline foods, such as leafy greens, cucumbers, celery, watermelon, and certain nuts and seeds, can help balance the pH of urine. On the other hand, acidic foods like citrus fruits, cranberries, and vinegar can increase the acidity of urine and potentially worsen IC symptoms.

- Individualized Approach: It is essential to recognize that the dietary triggers and responses to specific foods can vary among individuals with IC. While there are general guidelines for an anti-inflammatory IC diet, each person may have unique tolerances and sensitivities. It is crucial to adopt an individualized approach to identify personal trigger foods and tailor the diet accordingly.

It's important to note that dietary modifications alone

may not completely eliminate inflammation or resolve IC symptoms. IC is a complex condition, and a multimodal approach that combines dietary changes with other treatment strategies is often necessary for optimal symptom management. This may include medications, bladder instillations, physical therapy, stress management techniques, and lifestyle modifications.

When making dietary changes for IC, it is advisable to work closely with a healthcare professional or a registered dietitian who specializes in IC or urological conditions. They can provide personalized guidance, monitor progress, and help ensure that the diet remains balanced and nutritionally adequate.

In summary, inflammation plays a significant role in interstitial cystitis, contributing to bladder irritation and the development of symptoms. By adopting an anti-inflammatory diet and avoiding trigger foods, individuals with IC can help reduce inflammation levels and alleviate symptoms. Incorporating anti-inflammatory foods rich in antioxidants, omega-3 fatty acids, and phytochemicals can be beneficial. Hydration, maintaining an alkaline urine pH, and an individualized approach based on personal tolerances are also essential. However, it is crucial to recognize that dietary modifications should be part of a comprehensive treatment plan, and a healthcare professional's guidance is recommended to ensure a balanced approach to manage IC symptoms effectively.

Common triggers and irritants for IC patients

For individuals with interstitial cystitis (IC), certain triggers and irritants can exacerbate symptoms and lead to increased bladder inflammation and discomfort. While triggers can vary from person to person, there are several common culprits that are known to provoke IC symptoms. It's important for individuals with IC to identify and avoid these triggers as part of their management plan. Here are some of the most common triggers and irritants for IC patients:

- Acidic Foods and Beverages: Acidic foods and beverages can irritate the bladder and worsen IC symptoms. Examples include citrus fruits (lemons, oranges, grapefruits), tomatoes, cranberries, pineapple, and their juices. Acidic condiments like vinegar and certain salad dressings should also be avoided.
- Spicy Foods: Spicy foods can be highly irritating to the bladder and may trigger IC symptoms.

Common culprits include chili peppers, hot sauces, cayenne pepper, and spicy seasonings. It's best to avoid these foods or use milder alternatives to add flavor to meals.

- Caffeine: Caffeinated beverages like coffee, tea, energy drinks, and soda can be bladder irritants and increase urinary frequency and urgency in individuals with IC. It is advisable to limit or eliminate caffeine intake to help manage symptoms.
- Alcohol: Alcoholic beverages, including beer, wine, and spirits, can worsen IC symptoms by irritating the bladder and increasing urinary frequency. It is best to avoid alcohol or consume it in moderation, based on individual tolerances.
- Carbonated Beverages: Carbonated drinks, such as soda and sparkling water, can cause bladder distention and exacerbate IC symptoms. The carbonation can put additional pressure on the bladder, leading to increased discomfort.
- Artificial Sweeteners: Artificial sweeteners, such as aspartame and sucralose, found in diet sodas, sugar-free candies, and certain processed foods, can be bladder irritants for some individuals with IC. It's important to read food labels and opt for natural sweeteners like stevia or moderate consumption of sugar.
- Certain Medications: Some medications, including certain antibiotics, pain relievers (such as aspirin and ibuprofen), and medications with high acidity, may worsen IC symptoms in certain individuals. It's important to consult with a healthcare professional or pharmacist about

potential medication triggers for IC.

- Urinary Irritants: Certain substances that come into contact with the urinary tract can irritate the bladder and worsen IC symptoms. This includes harsh soaps, bubble baths, scented hygiene products, and douches. Using mild, fragrance-free products and avoiding irritants is recommended.
- Stress and Emotional Upsets: While not a direct food trigger, stress and emotional upsets can significantly impact IC symptoms. Stress can trigger flares and exacerbate bladder symptoms. Implementing stress management techniques, such as relaxation exercises, mindfulness, and therapy, can be beneficial.
- Dehydration: Insufficient hydration can concentrate urine and irritate the bladder, leading to increased symptoms for individuals with IC. It is important to stay properly hydrated by drinking adequate amounts of water throughout the day.
- Certain Food Additives: Some individuals with IC may be sensitive to food additives such as monosodium glutamate (MSG), artificial flavors, and preservatives. It is advisable to read food labels and avoid foods containing these additives if they are known triggers.
- Acidic Medications: Some medications, particularly those with high acidity, can irritate the bladder and worsen IC symptoms. It is important to discuss medication options with a healthcare professional, and if necessary, explore alternative options that are better tolerated.
- Physical Activity and Exercise: Intense physical activity, particularly exercises that put pressure

on the pelvic area, can trigger IC symptoms in some individuals. High-impact activities like running, jumping, or vigorous exercise may increase urinary urgency, frequency, and discomfort. It is important to find a balance between staying active and avoiding activities that worsen IC symptoms. Low-impact exercises such as swimming, walking, or gentle yoga may be better tolerated.

It's important to note that triggers and irritants can vary from person to person. While the aforementioned triggers are commonly reported by individuals with IC, each individual may have unique sensitivities and tolerances. It is crucial for individuals with IC to keep a detailed diary of their symptoms and potential triggers to identify personal triggers accurately. This can help guide them in making informed decisions about their diet, lifestyle choices, and overall management of IC.

In addition to identifying triggers, it is equally important for individuals with IC to focus on overall bladder health and practice self-care. This includes practicing good bladder habits, such as emptying the bladder regularly, avoiding holding urine for extended periods, and maintaining proper hygiene. Implementing stress management techniques, getting sufficient rest, and engaging in relaxation exercises can also help reduce the overall impact of triggers on IC symptoms.

Working closely with a healthcare professional, such as a urologist or a pelvic floor therapist, can provide valuable guidance and support in managing IC triggers. They can help identify individual triggers, provide dietary recommendations, suggest suitable medications, and develop a comprehensive treatment plan to address IC symptoms effectively.

In conclusion, understanding and avoiding triggers and irritants is an essential aspect of managing interstitial cystitis (IC). By identifying and avoiding common triggers such as acidic foods and beverages, spicy foods, caffeine, alcohol, artificial sweeteners, and certain medications, individuals with IC can help minimize bladder irritation and reduce symptom exacerbation. It is also important to pay attention to personal sensitivities and keep a diary to identify unique triggers. Adopting a holistic approach that includes lifestyle modifications, stress management, and good bladder habits can further contribute to overall symptom management and improved quality of life for individuals with IC.

IC Diet Guidelines

Overview of food groups and their impact on IC symptoms

When it comes to managing interstitial cystitis (IC) symptoms, understanding the impact of different food groups is crucial. While triggers can vary from person to person, certain food groups have been found to affect IC symptoms more than others. By paying attention to these food groups and making informed dietary choices, individuals with IC can potentially alleviate symptoms and improve their overall well-being. Here is an overview of different food groups and their potential impact on IC symptoms:

- Acidic Foods: Acidic foods can irritate the bladder lining and worsen IC symptoms. Examples of acidic foods include citrus fruits (lemons, oranges, grapefruits), tomatoes, cranberries, pineapples, and their juices. These foods contain compounds that can trigger inflammation and increase urinary frequency and urgency in individuals with IC. It is advisable to minimize or avoid these acidic foods if they are identified as triggers.

- Spicy Foods: Spicy foods, such as chili peppers, hot sauces, cayenne pepper, and spicy seasonings, can be highly irritating to the bladder. The capsaicin found in spicy foods can stimulate the release of substances that trigger inflammation and exacerbate IC symptoms. It is recommended to avoid or limit the consumption of spicy foods.
- Caffeine: Caffeinated beverages like coffee, tea, energy drinks, and soda can be bladder irritants and worsen IC symptoms. Caffeine is a diuretic that increases urinary frequency and can contribute to bladder irritation and discomfort. It is advisable to reduce or eliminate caffeine intake to help manage IC symptoms effectively.
- Alcohol: Alcoholic beverages, including beer, wine, and spirits, can irritate the bladder and increase urinary frequency and urgency in individuals with IC. Alcohol can also act as a diuretic and lead to dehydration, which can further exacerbate symptoms. It is best to limit or avoid alcohol consumption.
- Artificial Sweeteners: Artificial sweeteners, such as aspartame and sucralose, found in diet sodas, sugar-free candies, and certain processed foods, can be bladder irritants for some individuals with IC. These sweeteners may trigger bladder symptoms and should be avoided or consumed in moderation. Natural sweeteners like stevia or moderate amounts of sugar may be better tolerated alternatives.
- Dairy Products: Dairy products, particularly those high in fat, can potentially worsen IC symptoms for some individuals. The high fat content

may contribute to inflammation and bladder irritation. It is recommended to opt for low-fat or non-dairy alternatives like almond milk, coconut milk, or lactose-free products if dairy triggers symptoms.

- Gluten: While not directly linked to IC, some individuals with IC may have sensitivities to gluten or experience an overlap of symptoms with gluten-related conditions, such as celiac disease or gluten sensitivity. In such cases, avoiding gluten-containing grains like wheat, barley, and rye may be beneficial.
- Processed and Refined Foods: Processed and refined foods often contain artificial additives, preservatives, and high levels of sodium. These additives can trigger inflammation and contribute to IC symptoms. Opting for whole, unprocessed foods and preparing meals from scratch can help reduce exposure to these potential triggers.
- Anti-Inflammatory Foods: On the other hand, there are food groups that can help reduce inflammation and alleviate IC symptoms. Incorporating anti-inflammatory foods into the diet, such as fruits and vegetables rich in antioxidants, omega-3 fatty acids from sources like fatty fish, nuts, and seeds, can be beneficial for individuals with IC. Whole grains, lean proteins, and healthy fats like olive oil also contribute to an overall anti-inflammatory diet.

It's important to remember that while certain food groups are commonly associated with triggering or alleviating IC symptoms, each person's experience can be unique. It is essential to pay attention to individual sensitivities and responses to different food groups. Keeping a food diary and tracking symptoms can help identify specific triggers for each person.

In addition to the impact of specific food groups, it is also important to consider the overall balance and quality of the diet. Maintaining a well-rounded diet that includes a variety of nutrient-dense foods is beneficial for overall health and may help manage IC symptoms. This includes incorporating lean proteins, whole grains, fruits, vegetables, and healthy fats.

Furthermore, hydration is crucial for individuals with IC. Drinking an adequate amount of water throughout the day helps dilute urine and reduce bladder irritation. It is important to note that excessive fluid intake can also lead to increased urinary frequency, so finding a balance is key.

While making dietary modifications is a valuable step in managing IC symptoms, it is not a one-size-fits-all approach. Consulting with a healthcare professional or a registered dietitian who specializes in IC or urological conditions can provide personalized guidance and support. They can help identify individual triggers, develop a tailored dietary plan, and ensure that nutritional needs are met.

In conclusion, understanding the impact of different food groups on IC symptoms is important for individuals seeking to manage their condition effectively. Avoiding or limiting acidic foods, spicy foods, caffeine, alcohol, artificial sweeteners, and potentially triggering dairy or gluten products may help alleviate symptoms for many people. Conversely, incorporating anti-inflammatory foods and maintaining a well-balanced diet can support overall bladder health. It is essential to listen to the body, keep a food diary, and work with healthcare professionals to identify personal triggers and develop a customized approach to managing IC symptoms through dietary choices.

IC-friendly foods: a comprehensive list of safe options

When managing interstitial cystitis (IC), incorporating IC-friendly foods into your diet can help alleviate symptoms and support bladder health. While individual tolerances may vary, the following is a comprehensive list of commonly well-tolerated foods for many individuals with IC:

- Low-Acid Fruits: Opt for low-acid fruits like pears, melons (watermelon, cantaloupe, honeydew), bananas, and apples (in moderation). These fruits are less likely to irritate the bladder.
- Non-Acidic Vegetables: Choose non-acidic vegetables such as leafy greens (spinach, kale, lettuce), carrots, squash, sweet potatoes, cucumbers, and green beans. These vegetables are generally well-tolerated and provide essential nutrients.
- Lean Proteins: Include lean protein sources such as skinless poultry (chicken, turkey), fish (salmon, cod, tilapia), eggs, and tofu. These options provide important amino acids without excess fat or potential irritants.
- Whole Grains: Opt for whole grains like quinoa, brown rice, oats, and gluten-free grains (if tolerated). These grains offer fiber and nutrients while avoiding potential triggers.
- Healthy Fats: Incorporate healthy fats like olive oil, avocados, and small portions of nuts and seeds (if tolerated). These fats provide essential nutrients and can be beneficial for overall health.
- Herbal Teas: Enjoy herbal teas like chamomile, peppermint, and ginger tea. These beverages are

often soothing to the bladder and can provide comfort.

- Non-Citrus Juices: If you crave a fruit juice, try non-citrus options like pear juice or diluted apple juice. These options are generally better tolerated than highly acidic citrus juices.
- Dairy Alternatives: If dairy triggers symptoms, choose lactose-free or non-dairy alternatives like almond milk, coconut milk, or oat milk. Ensure that they do not contain additional additives or sweeteners.
- Water: Staying well-hydrated is essential for bladder health. Drink plenty of water throughout the day to maintain hydration and promote flushing of the urinary system.
- Fresh Herbs and Spices: Flavor your meals with fresh herbs and spices like basil, oregano, rosemary, thyme, and cinnamon. These additions can enhance taste without contributing to bladder irritation.
- Alternative Sweeteners: If needed, use alternative sweeteners like stevia or small amounts of sugar (if tolerated) to add sweetness to dishes or beverages. Avoid artificial sweeteners, which may trigger symptoms for some individuals.
- IC-Friendly Condiments: Choose IC-friendly condiments such as low-acid salad dressings (made with safe ingredients), mild mustards, and homemade sauces with IC-friendly ingredients.

Remember, it's important to listen to your body and keep a food diary to identify any personal triggers or sensitivities.

Additionally, portion sizes and overall balance remain key factors in maintaining a healthy diet. Consulting with a healthcare professional or a registered dietitian who specializes in IC can provide further guidance and tailor the diet to your specific needs.

While this list provides a starting point, individual responses may vary. It's important to find what works best for you and make adjustments based on your own tolerances and preferences.

Foods to avoid: a detailed list of common triggers

When managing interstitial cystitis (IC), it is important to be aware of common food triggers that can exacerbate symptoms. While triggers can vary from person to person, the following is a detailed list of commonly reported foods and ingredients that individuals with IC may want to avoid:

- Citrus Fruits: Oranges, lemons, grapefruits, and other citrus fruits are highly acidic and can irritate the bladder. It is best to avoid or limit consumption of these fruits and their juices.
- Tomatoes and Tomato-Based Products: Tomatoes

contain high levels of acid, which can be bothersome for individuals with IC. Avoid or minimize the consumption of tomatoes, tomato sauce, and tomato-based products.

- Spicy Foods: Spices like chili powder, cayenne pepper, and hot sauces can trigger bladder irritation and worsen IC symptoms. Limit or avoid spicy foods and seasonings.
- Caffeine: Caffeinated beverages such as coffee, tea, energy drinks, and soda can increase urinary frequency and urgency. Reduce or eliminate caffeine intake to help manage IC symptoms.
- Alcohol: Alcoholic beverages, including beer, wine, and spirits, can irritate the bladder and worsen IC symptoms. It is best to limit or avoid alcohol consumption.
- Carbonated Beverages: Carbonated drinks, including sparkling water and sodas, can lead to increased bladder pressure and discomfort. Limit or avoid carbonated beverages.
- Artificial Sweeteners: Artificial sweeteners like aspartame, saccharin, and sucralose found in diet sodas, sugar-free candies, and certain processed foods may trigger bladder symptoms. Avoid or minimize the consumption of foods and drinks containing these sweeteners.
- Highly Acidic Foods: Apart from citrus fruits, other highly acidic foods to avoid include pineapple, cranberries, sour cherries, and their juices. These acidic foods can irritate the bladder lining and worsen symptoms.
- High-Fat Foods: Foods high in fat, such as fried foods, fatty cuts of meat, and full-fat dairy

products, can contribute to inflammation and bladder irritation. Choose leaner protein sources and low-fat or non-dairy alternatives.

- Processed and Artificially Preserved Foods: Processed foods often contain additives, preservatives, and high levels of sodium, which can trigger inflammation and aggravate IC symptoms. Opt for whole, unprocessed foods whenever possible.
- Onions and Garlic: While not triggers for everyone, some individuals with IC may find that onions and garlic can cause bladder irritation. Pay attention to your own sensitivities and limit these ingredients if necessary.
- Certain Spices and Condiments: Some spices and condiments, such as black pepper, vinegar, mustard, and mayonnaise, can be irritating to the bladder. Consider using milder alternatives or minimizing their use.
- Artificial Colors and Flavors: Artificial food colorings and flavors, commonly found in processed snacks, candies, and drinks, can potentially trigger symptoms for individuals with IC. Opt for natural alternatives whenever possible.

It is important to note that triggers can be individualized, and what affects one person may not affect another. Keeping a detailed food diary and paying attention to personal reactions can help identify specific triggers. Consulting with a healthcare professional or a registered dietitian who specializes in IC can provide further guidance and support in managing your diet and identifying triggers that are specific to you.

SUGGEST A 7 DAYS MEAL PLAN FOR IC PATIENT

Here's a sample 7-day meal plan for individuals with interstitial cystitis (IC). Remember, individual tolerances may vary, so feel free to adjust the plan based on your personal needs and preferences:

Day 1:

- Breakfast: Oatmeal made with water or almond milk, topped with fresh blueberries and a drizzle of honey.
- Snack: A small handful of unsalted almonds.
- Lunch: Grilled chicken breast with steamed carrots and quinoa.
- Snack: Sliced cucumber with hummus.
- Dinner: Baked salmon with roasted asparagus and a side of brown rice.
- Dessert: A serving of vanilla coconut milk yogurt.

Day 2:

- Breakfast: Scrambled eggs with spinach and cherry tomatoes, served with a side of gluten-free toast.
- Snack: A banana.
- Lunch: Mixed greens salad with grilled shrimp,

avocado, and a lemon-tahini dressing.

- Snack: Rice cakes with almond butter.
- Dinner: Turkey meatballs with zucchini noodles and marinara sauce (using low-acid tomatoes).
- Dessert: Sliced strawberries with a dollop of coconut cream.

Day 3:

- Breakfast: Quinoa breakfast bowl with diced peaches, walnuts, and a sprinkle of cinnamon.
- Snack: Carrot sticks with a small portion of guacamole.
- Lunch: Lentil soup with a side of mixed greens salad.
- Snack: Greek yogurt with a drizzle of honey.
- Dinner: Grilled chicken with steamed green beans and sweet potato mash.
- Dessert: Baked cinnamon apples with a sprinkle of coconut flakes.

Day 4:

- Breakfast: Gluten-free pancakes topped with sliced bananas and a drizzle of maple syrup.
- Snack: A handful of blueberries.
- Lunch: Quinoa salad with roasted vegetables (such as bell peppers, zucchini, and eggplant) and feta cheese.
- Snack: Rice crackers with a side of hummus.
- Dinner: Baked cod with lemon-dill sauce, served with sautéed spinach and brown rice.
- Dessert: A small piece of dark chocolate.

Day 5:

- Breakfast: Chia seed pudding made with almond milk, topped with sliced strawberries and crushed almonds.
- Snack: Sliced bell peppers with a side of Greek yogurt dip.
- Lunch: Grilled tofu stir-fry with a variety of colorful vegetables and gluten-free soy sauce.
- Snack: Rice cakes with cashew butter.
- Dinner: Baked chicken breast with roasted Brussels sprouts and quinoa.
- Dessert: Sliced mango with a sprinkle of shredded coconut.

Day 6:

- Breakfast: Vegetable omelette (using non-irritating veggies like spinach, mushrooms, and bell peppers) with a side of gluten-free toast.
- Snack: A small handful of grapes.
- Lunch: Quinoa and black bean salad with diced tomatoes, cucumbers, and a lime-cilantro dressing.
- Snack: Celery sticks with almond butter.
- Dinner: Grilled shrimp skewers with grilled zucchini and brown rice.
- Dessert: A serving of coconut milk-based ice cream.

Day 7:

- Breakfast: Gluten-free overnight oats with almond milk, topped with sliced peaches and a sprinkle of cinnamon.
- Snack: A small portion of mixed nuts.
- Lunch: Spinach salad with grilled chicken,

strawberries, almonds, and a balsamic vinaigrette.
- Snack: Sliced pear with a side of Greek yogurt.
- Dinner: Baked turkey breast with steamed broccoli and quinoa.
- Dessert: Baked cinnamon pears with a drizzle of honey.

Remember to stay well hydrated throughout the day by drinking plenty of water. You can also incorporate IC-friendly beverages such as herbal teas, diluted fruit juices (non-citrus), and coconut water.

It's important to note that this sample meal plan is a general guide and should be adapted to your personal preferences, dietary needs, and individual tolerances. Consider working with a registered dietitian who specializes in IC or a healthcare professional for personalized guidance.

When following an IC meal plan, keep in mind the importance of portion control and mindful eating. Listening to your body and paying attention to how certain foods make you feel is key to managing IC symptoms effectively.

Additionally, it is essential to maintain a balanced and

nutritious diet by including a variety of nutrient-dense foods. This includes incorporating lean proteins, whole grains, fruits, vegetables, and healthy fats. Aim to choose organic, fresh, and minimally processed ingredients whenever possible.

Remember that managing IC involves a holistic approach, including stress management, adequate sleep, and regular physical activity. It's also important to consult with a healthcare professional or a registered dietitian to address any specific dietary concerns or questions you may have.

By following an IC-friendly meal plan and making informed choices about your diet, you can support bladder health, minimize symptoms, and improve your overall well-being.

CHAPTER TWO

Breakfast options:

Oatmeal with blueberries and honey

Ingredients:

- 1/2 cup rolled oats
- 1 cup water or almond milk (unsweetened)
- 1/2 cup fresh blueberries
- 1 tablespoon honey (adjust according to taste)
- Optional toppings: sliced almonds, chia seeds, or a sprinkle of cinnamon

Instructions:

- In a small saucepan, bring the water or almond milk to a gentle boil.
- Add the rolled oats to the boiling liquid and reduce the heat to low. Stir well to combine.
- Let the oats simmer for about 5 minutes, stirring occasionally, until they reach your desired consistency. If you prefer thicker oatmeal, you can simmer for a bit longer.
- Once the oatmeal reaches your desired consistency, remove the saucepan from the heat.
- Gently fold in the fresh blueberries, reserving a few for topping.
- Allow the oatmeal to sit for a minute or two to let the blueberries soften slightly.

- Transfer the oatmeal to a serving bowl.
- Drizzle the honey over the oatmeal and give it a gentle stir to incorporate the sweetness.
- If desired, top the oatmeal with the reserved fresh blueberries and any optional toppings like sliced almonds, chia seeds, or a sprinkle of cinnamon.
- Serve the oatmeal warm and enjoy!

Scrambled eggs with spinach and cherry tomatoes.

Ingredients:

- 2 large eggs
- 1 cup fresh spinach leaves
- 1/2 cup cherry tomatoes, halved
- Salt and pepper to taste
- Olive oil or cooking spray for greasing the pan
- Optional toppings: crumbled feta cheese, chopped herbs (such as parsley or chives)

Instructions:

- Crack the eggs into a small bowl and whisk them until well beaten. Season with salt and pepper according to your taste preference.
- Heat a non-stick skillet over medium heat. Lightly grease the skillet with olive oil or cooking spray.
- Add the fresh spinach leaves to the skillet and sauté for 1-2 minutes until wilted.
- Add the cherry tomatoes to the skillet and cook for another minute, just until they soften slightly.

- Reduce the heat to low and pour the beaten eggs into the skillet, ensuring they cover the spinach and cherry tomatoes evenly.
- Gently scramble the eggs with a spatula, stirring occasionally, until they reach your desired level of doneness. Some prefer softer, more moist scrambled eggs, while others prefer them well cooked.
- Once the eggs are cooked to your liking, remove the skillet from the heat.
- Transfer the scrambled eggs with spinach and cherry tomatoes to a plate or bowl.
- If desired, sprinkle crumbled feta cheese and chopped herbs over the eggs for added flavor and garnish.
- Serve the scrambled eggs warm as a delicious and nutritious breakfast or brunch option.

Quinoa breakfast bowl with peaches, walnuts, and cinnamon.

Ingredients:

- 1/2 cup cooked quinoa
- 1 ripe peach, sliced
- 2 tablespoons chopped walnuts
- 1/2 teaspoon ground cinnamon
- 1 tablespoon honey or maple syrup (optional, for sweetness)
- Splash of almond milk (optional, for added creaminess)

Instructions:

- Start by cooking the quinoa according to the package instructions. Once cooked, let it cool slightly before using it in the breakfast bowl.
- In a bowl, add the cooked quinoa as the base.
- Arrange the sliced peaches on top of the quinoa.
- Sprinkle the chopped walnuts over the peaches.
- Dust the entire bowl with ground cinnamon for a warm and cozy flavor.
- If desired, drizzle honey or maple syrup over the ingredients to add sweetness. Adjust the amount based on your preference.
- For added creaminess, you can also pour a splash of almond milk over the bowl.
- Give the ingredients a gentle stir to combine everything evenly.
- Enjoy the quinoa breakfast bowl immediately, savoring the delightful combination of flavors and textures.

Gluten-free pancakes with bananas and maple syrup.

Ingredients:

- 1 cup gluten-free all-purpose flour
- 2 tablespoons sugar (or sweetener of your choice)
- 1 teaspoon baking powder
- 1/2 teaspoon baking soda
- 1/4 teaspoon salt
- 1 cup buttermilk (or dairy-free alternative)

- 1 large egg
- 2 tablespoons melted butter (or dairy-free alternative)
- Sliced bananas for topping
- Maple syrup for serving

Instructions:

- In a mixing bowl, whisk together the gluten-free all-purpose flour, sugar, baking powder, baking soda, and salt.
- In a separate bowl, whisk together the buttermilk (or dairy-free alternative) and the egg until well combined.
- Pour the wet ingredients into the dry ingredients and mix until just combined. Be careful not to overmix, as it can result in tough pancakes.
- Stir in the melted butter (or dairy-free alternative) into the pancake batter.
- Heat a non-stick skillet or griddle over medium heat. Lightly grease the surface with cooking spray or a small amount of butter.
- Spoon about 1/4 cup of batter onto the skillet for each pancake. Spread the batter slightly with the back of the spoon to form a round shape.
- Cook the pancakes until bubbles start to form on the surface, then flip them carefully with a spatula. Cook for an additional 1-2 minutes until golden brown on both sides.
- Transfer the cooked pancakes to a serving plate.
- Top the pancakes with sliced bananas.
- Drizzle the stack of pancakes with maple syrup.
- Serve the gluten-free pancakes with bananas and maple syrup while they're still warm.

Chia seed pudding with strawberries and crushed almonds.

Ingredients:

- 3 tablespoons chia seeds
- 1 cup unsweetened almond milk (or any other milk of your choice)
- 1 tablespoon maple syrup or honey (adjust according to sweetness preference)
- 1/2 teaspoon vanilla extract
- Fresh strawberries, sliced
- Crushed almonds for topping

Instructions:

- In a bowl or mason jar, combine the chia seeds, almond milk, maple syrup or honey, and vanilla extract.
- Stir the mixture well to ensure the chia seeds are evenly distributed and not clumped together.
- Let the mixture sit for about 5 minutes and then stir again to prevent clumping.
- Cover the bowl or jar and refrigerate for at least 2 hours, or overnight, to allow the chia seeds to absorb the liquid and thicken.
- Once the chia seed pudding has set and reached a thick, pudding-like consistency, give it a good stir to break up any clumps.
- Spoon the chia seed pudding into serving bowls or glasses.
- Top the pudding with sliced strawberries and a

sprinkle of crushed almonds.
- Serve the chia seed pudding with strawberries and crushed almonds chilled.

Vegetable omelette with gluten-free toast.

Ingredients:

- 3 large eggs
- 2 tablespoons milk (dairy or non-dairy)
- Salt and pepper to taste
- 1 tablespoon olive oil
- 1/4 cup diced bell peppers (any color)
- 1/4 cup diced onions
- 1/4 cup sliced mushrooms
- Handful of baby spinach leaves
- Optional toppings: shredded cheese, chopped herbs (such as parsley or chives)
- 2 slices of gluten-free bread

Instructions:

- In a bowl, whisk together the eggs, milk, salt, and pepper until well combined.
- Heat olive oil in a non-stick skillet over medium heat.
- Add the diced bell peppers, onions, and mushrooms to the skillet. Sauté until the vegetables are softened and slightly caramelized.
- Add the baby spinach leaves to the skillet and cook until wilted.
- Reduce the heat to low and pour the beaten egg mixture over the sautéed vegetables in the skillet.

- Allow the eggs to cook undisturbed for a minute or two until the edges start to set.
- Gently lift the edges of the omelette with a spatula and tilt the skillet to allow the uncooked eggs to flow to the edges.
- Continue cooking the omelette until it is mostly set but still slightly runny on top.
- If desired, sprinkle shredded cheese and chopped herbs over half of the omelette.
- Fold the other half of the omelette over the cheese and herbs, creating a half-moon shape.
- Cook for an additional minute to melt the cheese and finish cooking the omelette.
- Meanwhile, toast the gluten-free bread slices until golden brown.
- Cut the omelette in half and transfer each portion to a plate.
- Serve the vegetable omelette with gluten-free toast on the side.

Gluten-free overnight oats with peaches and cinnamon.

Ingredients:

- 1/2 cup gluten-free rolled oats
- 1/2 cup almond milk (or any other milk of your choice)
- 1/4 cup Greek yogurt (or dairy-free alternative)
- 1 tablespoon chia seeds
- 1 tablespoon honey or maple syrup (adjust according to sweetness preference)

- 1/2 teaspoon ground cinnamon
- 1 ripe peach, sliced
- Optional toppings: sliced almonds, additional cinnamon, or a drizzle of honey

Instructions:

- In a mason jar or container with a lid, combine the rolled oats, almond milk, Greek yogurt, chia seeds, honey or maple syrup, and ground cinnamon.
- Stir the mixture well until all the ingredients are thoroughly combined.
- Add the sliced peaches to the mixture and gently stir to distribute them evenly.
- Seal the jar or container with the lid and refrigerate overnight, or for at least 4 hours, to allow the oats to absorb the liquid and soften.
- In the morning, give the overnight oats a good stir to ensure the ingredients are well mixed.
- If desired, you can add a splash of additional almond milk to adjust the consistency.
- Transfer the overnight oats to a serving bowl.
- Top the oats with any optional toppings such as sliced almonds, an extra sprinkle of cinnamon, or a drizzle of honey.
- Serve the gluten-free overnight oats with peaches and cinnamon chilled.

Snack options:

Handful of unsalted almonds.

Instructions:

- Take a handful of unsalted almonds, approximately 1/4 cup, and place them in a dry skillet or frying pan.
- Heat the skillet over medium heat and gently toast the almonds for about 3-5 minutes, stirring occasionally. Keep an eye on them to prevent burning.
- Once the almonds are lightly toasted, remove them from the heat and transfer them to a bowl.
- Allow the almonds to cool for a few minutes until they are safe to handle.
- Enjoy the handful of unsalted almonds as a delicious and wholesome snack.

Sliced cucumber with hummus.

Ingredients:

- 1 large cucumber
- 1 cup hummus (your choice of flavor)
- Optional toppings: paprika, chopped fresh herbs (such as parsley or dill), extra virgin olive oil

Instructions:

- Wash the cucumber thoroughly under cold water and pat it dry with a kitchen towel.
- Using a sharp knife or a mandoline slicer, slice the cucumber into thin rounds or sticks. You can leave the skin on or peel it based on your preference.
- Arrange the sliced cucumber on a serving platter or plate.

- In a separate bowl, scoop out the desired amount of hummus. You can use store-bought hummus or prepare homemade hummus using your preferred recipe.
- Place the bowl of hummus next to the sliced cucumber on the serving platter.
- If desired, you can sprinkle a pinch of paprika over the hummus for added flavor and visual appeal.
- Optional: Garnish the plate with chopped fresh herbs, such as parsley or dill, for a burst of freshness.
- Drizzle a small amount of extra virgin olive oil over the hummus for a touch of richness, if desired.
- Serve the sliced cucumber with hummus immediately as a refreshing and nutritious snack.

Small handful of blueberries.

Ingredients

- ¼ cup of fresh blueberry

Instructions:

- Take a small handful of fresh blueberries, approximately 1/4 to 1/2 cup, and place them in a bowl or a serving dish.
- Rinse the blueberries under cold water and gently pat them dry with a paper towel.
- Arrange the blueberries in the bowl, making sure they are evenly distributed.
- You can enjoy the blueberries as is, savoring their

natural sweetness and juiciness.

- Alternatively, if you'd like to add some extra flavor, consider sprinkling a small amount of granulated sugar or a drizzle of honey over the blueberries.
- For a tangy twist, squeeze a little fresh lemon juice over the blueberries.
- If desired, you can also sprinkle a pinch of cinnamon or a touch of vanilla extract over the blueberries for added depth of flavor.
- Gently toss the blueberries to coat them in the desired seasoning, being careful not to crush the delicate berries.
- Serve the small handful of blueberries as a refreshing and nutritious snack.

Carrot sticks with guacamole.

Ingredients:

- 2 large carrots, peeled and cut into sticks
- 2 ripe avocados
- 1 small tomato, diced
- 1/4 cup finely chopped red onion
- 1 clove garlic, minced
- Juice of 1 lime
- 2 tablespoons chopped fresh cilantro
- Salt and pepper to taste

Instructions:

- Peel the carrots and cut them into sticks of your desired size. Set them aside.

- Slice the avocados in half and remove the pits. Scoop out the flesh into a bowl.
- Mash the avocados using a fork until smooth and creamy.
- Add the diced tomato, chopped red onion, minced garlic, lime juice, and chopped cilantro to the bowl with the mashed avocados.
- Mix all the ingredients together until well combined.
- Season the guacamole with salt and pepper to taste. Adjust the seasoning according to your preference.
- Transfer the guacamole to a serving bowl.
- Arrange the carrot sticks on a plate or a platter.
- Serve the carrot sticks alongside the guacamole, allowing guests to dip the carrot sticks into the flavorful guacamole.

Rice cakes with almond butter.

Ingredients:

- Rice cakes (plain or flavored, according to your preference)
- Almond butter (smooth or crunchy, based on your preference)
- Optional toppings: Sliced bananas, drizzle of honey, sprinkle of cinnamon, chia seeds, or sliced almonds

Instructions:

- Take a rice cake and place it on a plate or a serving

dish.
- Spread a generous amount of almond butter evenly on top of the rice cake. You can use smooth or crunchy almond butter, depending on your texture preference.
- If desired, you can add additional toppings to enhance the flavor and texture of the rice cake. Some delicious options include sliced bananas, a drizzle of honey, a sprinkle of cinnamon, chia seeds, or sliced almonds.
- Repeat the process for as many rice cakes as you'd like to prepare.
- Serve the rice cakes with almond butter immediately.

Rice crackers with hummus.

Ingredients:

- Rice crackers (plain or flavored, according to your preference)
- Hummus (your choice of flavor)
- Optional toppings: Thinly sliced cucumbers, cherry tomatoes, fresh herbs (such as parsley or dill), or a drizzle of olive oil

Instructions:

- Take a rice cracker and place it on a serving plate or platter.
- Spoon a dollop of hummus onto the rice cracker. You can use classic hummus or experiment with different flavors like roasted red pepper or garlic.

- If desired, you can add additional toppings to enhance the flavor and presentation. Thinly sliced cucumbers, halved cherry tomatoes, or a sprinkle of fresh herbs like parsley or dill can add a pop of color and freshness. A drizzle of olive oil over the toppings can also provide an extra layer of flavor.
- Repeat the process for as many rice crackers as you'd like to prepare.
- Serve the rice crackers with hummus immediately.

Handful of grapes.

Ingredients:

- Handful of fresh grapes (any variety you prefer)
- Cheese cubes (such as cheddar, mozzarella, or goat cheese)
- Toothpicks or small skewers

Instructions:

- Wash the grapes under cold water and pat them dry with a paper towel.
- Prepare the cheese cubes by cutting them into bite-sized pieces that are similar in size to the grapes.
- Take a toothpick or a small skewer and thread a grape onto it.
- Follow with a cheese cube, piercing it through the center.
- Continue alternating between grapes and cheese cubes until the toothpick or skewer is full, leaving

enough space at the end to hold.
- Repeat the process to create additional grape and cheese skewers with the remaining grapes and cheese.
- Arrange the grape and cheese skewers on a serving platter or plate.
- Serve the grape and cheese skewers immediately as a delicious and refreshing snack.

Small portion of mixed nuts.

Ingredients:

- Small portion of mixed nuts (such as almonds, cashews, walnuts, peanuts, or pecans)
- Optional: Dried fruits (such as cranberries, raisins, or apricots)
- Optional: Dark chocolate chips or chunks
- Optional: Sprinkle of sea salt or your preferred seasoning

Instructions:

- Take a small portion of mixed nuts, approximately a handful, and place them in a bowl.
- If desired, add a handful of dried fruits to the bowl. Dried cranberries, raisins, or chopped apricots work well with mixed nuts.
- For a touch of indulgence, sprinkle in a handful of dark chocolate chips or chunks. The sweetness of the chocolate complements the nuts nicely.
- If you prefer a savory flavor, sprinkle a little sea salt or your preferred seasoning over the mixture.

- Gently toss the nuts, dried fruits, and any additional ingredients together until they are evenly combined.
- Serve the mixed nut snack mix in a small bowl or divide into individual portions for convenient snacking.

Lunch options:

Grilled chicken breast with steamed carrots and quinoa.

Ingredients:

- 2 boneless, skinless chicken breasts
- 2 cups baby carrots
- 1 cup quinoa
- 2 cups water or chicken broth
- Salt and pepper to taste
- Olive oil for grilling

Instructions:

- Preheat your grill to medium-high heat.
- Season the chicken breasts with salt and pepper on both sides.
- Lightly brush the grill grates with olive oil to prevent sticking.
- Place the seasoned chicken breasts on the grill and cook for about 6-8 minutes per side or until the internal temperature reaches 165°F (74°C). Cooking time may vary depending on the

thickness of the chicken breasts.

- While the chicken is grilling, prepare the steamed carrots and quinoa.
- In a saucepan, bring the water or chicken broth to a boil. Rinse the quinoa under cold water and add it to the boiling liquid.
- Reduce the heat to low, cover the saucepan, and let the quinoa simmer for about 15 minutes or until the liquid is absorbed and the quinoa is fluffy.
- In a separate pot, place the baby carrots and add enough water to cover them. Bring the water to a boil and then reduce the heat to medium-low. Cover the pot and steam the carrots for about 10-12 minutes or until they are tender.
- Once the chicken is cooked through, remove it from the grill and let it rest for a few minutes before slicing.
- Serve the grilled chicken breast alongside the steamed carrots and quinoa. You can season the carrots and quinoa with a sprinkle of salt and pepper if desired.
- Enjoy your delicious and nutritious grilled chicken breast with steamed carrots and quinoa!

Mixed greens salad with grilled shrimp and lemon-tahini dressing.

Ingredients:

For the Salad:

- 1 pound large shrimp, peeled and deveined

- 6 cups mixed salad greens (such as lettuce, spinach, arugula, or kale)
- 1 cup cherry tomatoes, halved
- 1 cucumber, sliced
- 1/4 red onion, thinly sliced
- Fresh herbs (such as parsley or dill), chopped (optional)
- Salt and pepper to taste

For the Lemon-Tahini Dressing:

- 2 tablespoons tahini
- Juice of 1 lemon
- 2 tablespoons olive oil
- 1 clove garlic, minced
- 1 tablespoon honey (optional, for sweetness)
- Salt and pepper to taste
- Water (as needed to thin out the dressing)

Instructions:

- Preheat your grill to medium-high heat.
- In a bowl, season the shrimp with salt and pepper. Toss to coat evenly.
- Grill the shrimp for about 2-3 minutes per side until they are pink and cooked through. Set them aside to cool slightly.
- In a large salad bowl, combine the mixed salad greens, cherry tomatoes, cucumber slices, and red onion. Add fresh herbs, if desired.
- In a separate small bowl, whisk together the tahini, lemon juice, olive oil, minced garlic, honey (if using), salt, and pepper until well combined.
- Gradually add water to the dressing while whisking until the desired consistency is

achieved. The dressing should be smooth and pourable.

- Pour the lemon-tahini dressing over the salad ingredients. Toss gently to coat the greens evenly.
- Divide the dressed salad onto serving plates or bowls.
- Arrange the grilled shrimp on top of the salad.
- Garnish with additional fresh herbs, if desired.
- Serve the mixed greens salad with grilled shrimp immediately, and enjoy!

Lentil soup with a side of mixed greens salad.

Ingredients:

For the Lentil Soup:

- 1 cup dried lentils (green or brown), rinsed
- 1 onion, diced
- 2 carrots, diced
- 2 celery stalks, diced
- 3 cloves garlic, minced
- 4 cups vegetable or chicken broth
- 1 can diced tomatoes (14 ounces)
- 1 teaspoon ground cumin
- 1 teaspoon ground coriander
- 1/2 teaspoon smoked paprika
- Salt and pepper to taste
- Olive oil for sautéing

For the Mixed Greens Salad:

- 4 cups mixed salad greens (such as lettuce, spinach, arugula, or kale)

- 1 cup cherry tomatoes, halved
- 1/2 cucumber, sliced
- 1/4 red onion, thinly sliced
- Optional toppings: Crumbled feta cheese, sliced almonds, or dried cranberries
- Salad dressing of your choice

Instructions:

For the Lentil Soup:

- In a large pot, heat olive oil over medium heat.
- Add the diced onion, carrots, and celery to the pot. Sauté for about 5 minutes until the vegetables start to soften.
- Add the minced garlic and sauté for an additional minute.
- Stir in the rinsed lentils, vegetable or chicken broth, diced tomatoes, cumin, coriander, smoked paprika, salt, and pepper.
- Bring the mixture to a boil, then reduce the heat to low. Cover the pot and let the soup simmer for about 30-40 minutes until the lentils are tender.
- Taste the soup and adjust the seasoning if needed.
- Serve the lentil soup hot and garnish with fresh herbs if desired.

For the Mixed Greens Salad:

- In a large salad bowl, combine the mixed salad greens, cherry tomatoes, cucumber slices, and red onion.
- Add any optional toppings you desire, such as crumbled feta cheese, sliced almonds, or dried cranberries.

- Drizzle your preferred salad dressing over the salad. Toss gently to coat the greens evenly.

To serve:

- Ladle the warm lentil soup into bowls.
- Serve each bowl of soup with a side of the mixed greens salad.

Quinoa salad with roasted vegetables and feta cheese.

Ingredients:

For the Quinoa Salad:

- 1 cup quinoa
- 2 cups water or vegetable broth
- 1 small eggplant, diced
- 1 zucchini, diced
- 1 red bell pepper, diced
- 1 yellow bell pepper, diced
- 1 red onion, sliced
- 3 tablespoons olive oil, divided
- 1 teaspoon dried herbs (such as thyme or oregano)
- Salt and pepper to taste
- 1/2 cup crumbled feta cheese
- Fresh parsley or basil, chopped (optional, for garnish)

For the Dressing:

- 3 tablespoons extra virgin olive oil
- 2 tablespoons lemon juice

- 1 garlic clove, minced
- 1 teaspoon Dijon mustard
- Salt and pepper to taste

Instructions:

- Preheat the oven to 400°F (200°C).
- In a fine-mesh strainer, rinse the quinoa under cold water. In a saucepan, combine the rinsed quinoa with water or vegetable broth. Bring to a boil, then reduce the heat to low, cover, and simmer for about 15-20 minutes until the quinoa is cooked and the liquid is absorbed. Fluff the quinoa with a fork and set it aside to cool.
- In a large mixing bowl, combine the diced eggplant, zucchini, bell peppers, and sliced red onion. Drizzle with 2 tablespoons of olive oil, sprinkle with dried herbs, salt, and pepper. Toss to coat the vegetables evenly.
- Spread the vegetables in a single layer on a baking sheet. Roast in the preheated oven for about 20-25 minutes until the vegetables are tender and slightly caramelized. Remove from the oven and let them cool slightly.
- In a small bowl, whisk together the extra virgin olive oil, lemon juice, minced garlic, Dijon mustard, salt, and pepper to make the dressing.
- In a large salad bowl, combine the cooked quinoa, roasted vegetables, and crumbled feta cheese.
- Drizzle the dressing over the quinoa salad and toss gently to coat all the ingredients.
- Taste and adjust the seasoning if needed.
- Garnish with fresh parsley or basil, if desired.
- Serve the quinoa salad with roasted vegetables

and feta cheese chilled or at room temperature.

Grilled tofu stir-fry with colorful vegetables and gluten-free soy sauce.

Ingredients:

For the Grilled Tofu:

- 1 block firm tofu
- 2 tablespoons gluten-free soy sauce
- 1 tablespoon sesame oil
- 1 tablespoon rice vinegar
- 1 teaspoon honey or maple syrup (optional, for sweetness)
- Salt and pepper to taste

For the Stir-Fry:

- 1 tablespoon olive oil
- 1 red bell pepper, thinly sliced
- 1 yellow bell pepper, thinly sliced
- 1 small broccoli head, florets separated
- 1 medium carrot, thinly sliced
- 1 cup sugar snap peas, ends trimmed
- 2 cloves garlic, minced
- 1-inch piece fresh ginger, grated
- 2 tablespoons gluten-free soy sauce
- 1 tablespoon rice vinegar
- 1 tablespoon honey or maple syrup (optional, for sweetness)
- Salt and pepper to taste
- Sesame seeds for garnish (optional)

Instructions:

For the Grilled Tofu:

- Drain the tofu and pat it dry with paper towels. Cut the tofu into bite-sized cubes.
- In a bowl, whisk together the gluten-free soy sauce, sesame oil, rice vinegar, honey or maple syrup (if using), salt, and pepper.
- Add the tofu cubes to the marinade and gently toss to coat. Let it marinate for about 15-20 minutes to allow the flavors to infuse.
- Preheat a grill pan or grill over medium-high heat.
- Place the marinated tofu cubes on the hot grill and cook for about 3-4 minutes per side until they are browned and slightly crispy. Remove from the grill and set aside.

For the Stir-Fry:

- Heat olive oil in a large skillet or wok over medium-high heat.
- Add the sliced bell peppers, broccoli florets, carrot slices, and sugar snap peas to the skillet. Stir-fry for about 3-4 minutes until the vegetables are crisp-tender.
- Add the minced garlic and grated ginger to the skillet. Stir-fry for an additional minute until fragrant.
- In a small bowl, whisk together the gluten-free soy sauce, rice vinegar, honey or maple syrup (if using), salt, and pepper.
- Pour the sauce over the vegetables in the skillet. Stir-fry for another 2-3 minutes until the

- vegetables are coated with the sauce and heated through.
- Add the grilled tofu cubes to the skillet and gently toss to combine with the vegetables.
- Taste and adjust the seasoning if needed.
- Remove from heat and transfer the grilled tofu stir-fry to a serving dish.
- Garnish with sesame seeds, if desired.

Quinoa and black bean salad with tomatoes, cucumbers, and lime-cilantro dressing.

Ingredients:

For the Quinoa and Black Bean Salad:

- 1 cup quinoa
- 2 cups water or vegetable broth
- 1 can black beans, rinsed and drained
- 1 cup cherry tomatoes, halved
- 1 cucumber, diced
- ¼ red onion, finely chopped
- ¼ cup chopped fresh cilantro
- Salt and pepper to taste

For the Lime-Cilantro Dressing:

- Juice of 2 limes
- 3 tablespoons extra virgin olive oil
- 1 tablespoon honey or maple syrup
- 1 clove garlic, minced
- ¼ cup chopped fresh cilantro
- Salt and pepper to taste

Instructions:

For the Quinoa and Black Bean Salad:

- Rinse the quinoa under cold water using a fine-mesh strainer.
- In a saucepan, combine the rinsed quinoa with water or vegetable broth. Bring to a boil, then reduce the heat to low, cover, and simmer for about 15-20 minutes until the quinoa is cooked and the liquid is absorbed. Fluff the quinoa with a fork and set it aside to cool.
- In a large mixing bowl, combine the cooked quinoa, black beans, cherry tomatoes, cucumber, red onion, and chopped cilantro.
- Season with salt and pepper to taste. Toss gently to combine all the ingredients.

For the Lime-Cilantro Dressing:

- In a small bowl, whisk together the lime juice, extra virgin olive oil, honey or maple syrup, minced garlic, chopped cilantro, salt, and pepper.
- Taste and adjust the seasoning if needed.

To Assemble:

- Pour the Lime-Cilantro Dressing over the quinoa and black bean salad.
- Gently toss the salad to coat all the ingredients with the dressing.
- Let the salad sit for about 10-15 minutes to allow the flavors to meld together.
- Serve the quinoa and black bean salad chilled or at room temperature.

Spinach salad with grilled chicken, strawberries, almonds, and balsamic vinaigrette.

Ingredients:

For the Grilled Chicken:

- 2 boneless, skinless chicken breasts
- 2 tablespoons olive oil
- 2 tablespoons balsamic vinegar
- 2 cloves garlic, minced
- Salt and pepper to taste

For the Spinach Salad:

- 6 cups fresh baby spinach leaves
- 1 cup sliced strawberries
- 1/2 cup sliced almonds
- 1/4 red onion, thinly sliced
- 1/4 cup crumbled feta cheese (optional)

For the Balsamic Vinaigrette:

- 1/4 cup balsamic vinegar
- 1/4 cup extra virgin olive oil
- 1 tablespoon honey or maple syrup
- 1 teaspoon Dijon mustard
- Salt and pepper to taste

Instructions:

For the Grilled Chicken:

- Preheat a grill or grill pan over medium-high heat.
- In a bowl, whisk together olive oil, balsamic vinegar, minced garlic, salt, and pepper.
- Place the chicken breasts in a shallow dish and pour the marinade over them, turning to coat both sides. Let it marinate for about 15-20 minutes.
- Grill the chicken breasts for about 6-8 minutes per side, or until cooked through and no longer pink in the center.
- Remove the chicken from the grill and let it rest for a few minutes. Slice the chicken into thin strips.

For the Spinach Salad:

- In a large salad bowl, combine the fresh baby spinach leaves, sliced strawberries, sliced almonds, and thinly sliced red onion.
- If desired, sprinkle crumbled feta cheese over the salad.

For the Balsamic Vinaigrette:

- In a small bowl, whisk together balsamic vinegar, extra virgin olive oil, honey or maple syrup, Dijon mustard, salt, and pepper.
- Taste and adjust the seasoning if needed.

To Assemble:

- Drizzle the Balsamic Vinaigrette over the spinach salad.

- Toss the salad gently to coat all the ingredients with the dressing.
- Top the salad with the grilled chicken slices.
- Serve the spinach salad with grilled chicken, strawberries, almonds, and balsamic vinaigrette immediately.

Dinner options:

Baked salmon with roasted asparagus and brown rice.

Ingredients:

For the Baked Salmon:

- 2 salmon fillets
- 2 tablespoons olive oil
- 1 tablespoon lemon juice
- 2 cloves garlic, minced
- Salt and pepper to taste

For the Roasted Asparagus:

- 1 bunch asparagus, trimmed
- 2 tablespoons olive oil
- Salt and pepper to taste

For the Brown Rice:

- 1 cup brown rice
- 2 cups water or vegetable broth
- Salt to taste

Instructions:

For the Baked Salmon:

- Preheat the oven to 375°F (190°C).
- Place the salmon fillets on a baking sheet lined with parchment paper.
- In a small bowl, whisk together the olive oil, lemon juice, minced garlic, salt, and pepper.
- Pour the marinade over the salmon fillets, making sure they are evenly coated.
- Bake the salmon in the preheated oven for about 12-15 minutes, or until cooked through and flaky.

For the Roasted Asparagus:

- Preheat the oven to 425°F (220°C).
- Place the trimmed asparagus on a baking sheet.
- Drizzle olive oil over the asparagus and season with salt and pepper.
- Toss the asparagus to ensure they are coated with oil and seasoning.
- Roast the asparagus in the preheated oven for about 10-12 minutes, or until tender and slightly crispy.

For the Brown Rice:

- Rinse the brown rice under cold water using a fine-mesh strainer.
- In a saucepan, combine the rinsed brown rice with water or vegetable broth and salt.
- Bring to a boil, then reduce the heat to low, cover, and simmer for about 45-50 minutes, or until the rice is tender and all the liquid is absorbed.

- Remove from heat and let it sit covered for 5 minutes. Fluff the rice with a fork before serving.

To Assemble:

- Divide the baked salmon fillets, roasted asparagus, and cooked brown rice among serving plates.
- Serve the baked salmon alongside the roasted asparagus and brown rice.

Turkey meatballs with zucchini noodles and low-acid

Ingredients:

For the Turkey Meatballs:

- 1 pound ground turkey
- 1/4 cup breadcrumbs (gluten-free if desired)
- 1/4 cup grated Parmesan cheese (optional)
- 1/4 cup finely chopped onion
- 2 cloves garlic, minced
- 1/4 cup chopped fresh parsley
- 1 teaspoon dried oregano
- 1/2 teaspoon salt
- 1/4 teaspoon black pepper
- 1 egg, beaten

For the Zucchini Noodles:

- 4 medium-sized zucchini
- 2 tablespoons olive oil
- Salt and pepper to taste

For the Low-Acid Tomato Sauce:

- 1 can (14 ounces) low-acid tomato sauce
- 1/4 cup tomato paste
- 2 cloves garlic, minced
- 1 teaspoon dried basil
- 1 teaspoon dried oregano
- 1/2 teaspoon dried thyme
- Salt and pepper to taste

Instructions:

For the Turkey Meatballs:

- Preheat the oven to 375°F (190°C).
- In a large mixing bowl, combine ground turkey, breadcrumbs, grated Parmesan cheese (if using), chopped onion, minced garlic, chopped parsley, dried oregano, salt, black pepper, and beaten egg.
- Mix all the ingredients together until well combined.
- Shape the mixture into small meatballs, about 1-1.5 inches in diameter.
- Place the meatballs on a baking sheet lined with parchment paper.
- Bake the meatballs in the preheated oven for about 20-25 minutes, or until cooked through and browned.

For the Zucchini Noodles:

- Trim the ends of the zucchini and spiralize them into noodles using a spiralizer.
- Heat olive oil in a large skillet over medium heat.
- Add the zucchini noodles to the skillet and sauté

for about 3-5 minutes, or until they are tender but still slightly crisp.
- Season with salt and pepper to taste.

For the Low-Acid Tomato Sauce:

- In a saucepan, combine the low-acid tomato sauce, tomato paste, minced garlic, dried basil, dried oregano, dried thyme, salt, and pepper.
- Stir well to combine all the ingredients.
- Cook the sauce over medium-low heat for about 10-15 minutes, allowing the flavors to meld together.

To Assemble:

- Place a serving of zucchini noodles on each plate.
- Top the zucchini noodles with a generous amount of low-acid tomato sauce.
- Arrange several turkey meatballs on top of the tomato sauce.
- Serve the turkey meatballs with zucchini noodles and low-acid tomato sauce hot.

Baked cod with lemon-dill sauce, served with sautéed spinach and brown rice.

Ingredients:

- For the Baked Cod:
- 4 cod fillets (about 6 ounces each)
- 2 tablespoons olive oil
- 2 tablespoons fresh lemon juice
- 2 cloves garlic, minced

- Salt and pepper to taste

For the Lemon-Dill Sauce:

- 1/2 cup plain Greek yogurt
- 1 tablespoon fresh lemon juice
- 1 tablespoon chopped fresh dill
- 1/2 teaspoon lemon zest
- Salt and pepper to taste

For the Sautéed Spinach:

- 1 tablespoon olive oil
- 2 cloves garlic, minced
- 8 cups fresh spinach leaves
- Salt and pepper to taste

For the Brown Rice:

- 1 cup brown rice
- 2 cups water or vegetable broth
- Salt to taste

Instructions:

For the Baked Cod:

- Preheat the oven to 400°F (200°C).
- Place the cod fillets in a baking dish lined with parchment paper.
- In a small bowl, whisk together olive oil, lemon juice, minced garlic, salt, and pepper.
- Pour the marinade over the cod fillets, making sure they are evenly coated.
- Bake the cod in the preheated oven for about 12-15 minutes, or until it flakes easily with a fork.

For the Lemon-Dill Sauce:

- In a small bowl, combine Greek yogurt, lemon juice, chopped fresh dill, lemon zest, salt, and pepper.
- Stir well to combine all the ingredients.
- Taste and adjust the seasoning if needed.

For the Sautéed Spinach:

- Heat olive oil in a large skillet over medium heat.
- Add minced garlic and sauté for about 1 minute, until fragrant.
- Add fresh spinach leaves to the skillet and sauté for about 2-3 minutes, or until wilted.
- Season with salt and pepper to taste.

For the Brown Rice:

- Rinse the brown rice under cold water using a fine-mesh strainer.
- In a saucepan, combine the rinsed brown rice with water or vegetable broth and salt.
- Bring to a boil, then reduce the heat to low, cover, and simmer for about 45-50 minutes, or until the rice is tender and all the liquid is absorbed.
- Remove from heat and let it sit covered for 5 minutes. Fluff the rice with a fork before serving.

To Assemble:

- Divide the baked cod fillets among serving plates.
- Drizzle each fillet with the lemon-dill sauce.
- Serve the cod with a side of sautéed

Baked chicken breast with roasted Brussels sprouts and quinoa.

Ingredients:

For the Baked Chicken Breast:

- 4 boneless, skinless chicken breasts
- 2 tablespoons olive oil
- 1 teaspoon garlic powder
- 1 teaspoon paprika
- 1/2 teaspoon salt
- 1/4 teaspoon black pepper

For the Roasted Brussels Sprouts:

1 pound Brussels sprouts, trimmed and halved

- 2 tablespoons olive oil
- 1 teaspoon garlic powder
- 1/2 teaspoon salt
- 1/4 teaspoon black pepper

For the Quinoa:

- 1 cup quinoa
- 2 cups water or chicken broth
- 1/2 teaspoon salt

Instructions:

For the Baked Chicken Breast:

- Preheat the oven to 425°F (220°C).

- Place the chicken breasts on a baking sheet lined with parchment paper.
- Drizzle olive oil over the chicken breasts and rub them evenly to coat.
- In a small bowl, combine garlic powder, paprika, salt, and black pepper.
- Sprinkle the spice mixture evenly over the chicken breasts, coating both sides.
- Bake the chicken in the preheated oven for about 20-25 minutes, or until the internal temperature reaches 165°F (74°C) and the chicken is cooked through.

For the Roasted Brussels Sprouts:

- Preheat the oven to 425°F (220°C).
- Place the halved Brussels sprouts on a baking sheet.
- Drizzle olive oil over the Brussels sprouts and toss to coat them evenly.
- Sprinkle garlic powder, salt, and black pepper over the Brussels sprouts, tossing to ensure they are evenly seasoned.
- Roast the Brussels sprouts in the preheated oven for about 20-25 minutes, or until they are tender and slightly caramelized.

For the Quinoa:

- Rinse the quinoa under cold water using a fine-mesh strainer.
- In a saucepan, combine the rinsed quinoa with water or chicken broth and salt.
- Bring to a boil, then reduce the heat to low, cover, and simmer for about 15-20 minutes, or until the

quinoa is fluffy and the liquid is absorbed.

- Remove from heat and let it sit covered for 5 minutes. Fluff the quinoa with a fork before serving.

To Assemble:

- Divide the baked chicken breasts among serving plates.
- Arrange a portion of roasted Brussels sprouts next to the chicken.
- Serve the chicken and Brussels sprouts with a side of cooked quinoa.

Grilled shrimp skewers with grilled zucchini and brown

Ingredients:

For the Grilled Shrimp Skewers:

- 1 pound large shrimp, peeled and deveined
- 2 tablespoons olive oil
- 2 cloves garlic, minced
- 1 tablespoon fresh lemon juice
- 1 teaspoon paprika
- 1/2 teaspoon salt
- 1/4 teaspoon black pepper
- Wooden skewers, soaked in water for 30 minutes

For the Grilled Zucchini:

- 2 medium-sized zucchini, sliced into 1/4-inch thick rounds
- 2 tablespoons olive oil
- 1 teaspoon dried oregano
- 1/2 teaspoon garlic powder
- 1/2 teaspoon salt
- 1/4 teaspoon black pepper

For the Brown Rice:

- 1 cup brown rice
- 2 cups water or vegetable broth
- 1/2 teaspoon salt

Instructions:

For the Grilled Shrimp Skewers:

- In a bowl, combine olive oil, minced garlic, lemon juice, paprika, salt, and black pepper.
- Add the peeled and deveined shrimp to the bowl and toss to coat them evenly with the marinade.
- Thread the shrimp onto the soaked wooden skewers.
- Preheat the grill to medium-high heat.
- Place the shrimp skewers on the grill and cook for about 2-3 minutes per side, or until the shrimp are pink and cooked through.

For the Grilled Zucchini:

- Preheat the grill to medium-high heat.
- In a bowl, combine olive oil, dried oregano, garlic powder, salt, and black pepper.
- Add the zucchini slices to the bowl and toss to coat

them evenly with the marinade.

- Place the zucchini slices directly on the grill grates and cook for about 3-4 minutes per side, or until they are tender and have grill marks.

For the Brown Rice:

- Rinse the brown rice under cold water using a fine-mesh strainer.
- In a saucepan, combine the rinsed brown rice with water or vegetable broth and salt.
- Bring to a boil, then reduce the heat to low, cover, and simmer for about 45-50 minutes, or until the rice is tender and all the liquid is absorbed.
- Remove from heat and let it sit covered for 5 minutes. Fluff the rice with a fork before serving.

To Assemble:

- Divide the grilled shrimp skewers among serving plates.
- Arrange a portion of grilled zucchini slices next to the shrimp.
- Serve the shrimp skewers and grilled zucchini with a side of cooked brown rice.

Baked turkey breast with steamed broccoli and quinoa.

Ingredients:

For the Baked Turkey Breast:

- 1.5 pounds turkey breast, boneless and skinless

- 2 tablespoons olive oil
- 1 teaspoon dried thyme
- 1 teaspoon dried rosemary
- 1 teaspoon garlic powder
- 1/2 teaspoon salt
- 1/4 teaspoon black pepper

For the Steamed Broccoli:

- 2 cups broccoli florets
- Water for steaming
- Pinch of salt

For the Quinoa:

- 1 cup quinoa
- 2 cups water or chicken broth
- 1/2 teaspoon salt

Instructions:

For the Baked Turkey Breast:

- Preheat the oven to 375°F (190°C).
- Place the turkey breast on a baking dish or roasting pan.
- Drizzle olive oil over the turkey breast, then rub it evenly to coat.
- In a small bowl, combine dried thyme, dried rosemary, garlic powder, salt, and black pepper.
- Sprinkle the herb mixture evenly over the turkey breast, patting it gently to adhere.
- Bake the turkey breast in the preheated oven for about 30-40 minutes, or until it reaches an internal temperature of 165°F (74°C) and is

cooked through.

- Let the turkey breast rest for a few minutes before slicing.

For the Steamed Broccoli:

- Fill a pot with water and bring it to a boil.
- Place the broccoli florets in a steamer basket or colander, and place it over the boiling water.
- Cover the pot and steam the broccoli for about 4-5 minutes, or until it is tender-crisp.
- Remove the steamed broccoli from the pot and sprinkle with a pinch of salt.

For the Quinoa:

- Rinse the quinoa under cold water using a fine-mesh strainer.
- In a saucepan, combine the rinsed quinoa with water or chicken broth and salt.
- Bring to a boil, then reduce the heat to low, cover, and simmer for about 15-20 minutes, or until the quinoa is fluffy and the liquid is absorbed.
- Remove from heat and let it sit covered for 5 minutes. Fluff the quinoa with a fork before serving.

To Assemble:

- Slice the baked turkey breast into thin slices.
- Divide the turkey slices among serving plates.
- Arrange a portion of steamed broccoli next to the turkey slices.
- Serve the turkey breast and steamed broccoli with a side of cooked quinoa.

Dessert options:

Vanilla coconut milk yogurt.

Ingredients:

- 2 cans (800 ml) full-fat coconut milk
- 2 tablespoons maple syrup or honey
- 2 teaspoons vanilla extract
- 2 teaspoons agar-agar powder (optional, for thickening)
- Yogurt starter culture or probiotic capsules (look for dairy-free options)
- Cheesecloth or nut milk bag
- Glass jars or containers for storage

Instructions:

- Start by sterilizing your equipment. Wash the glass jars or containers with hot, soapy water, and rinse them thoroughly. Alternatively, you can run them through a dishwasher cycle.
- In a large saucepan, pour the coconut milk and place it over medium heat. Warm the coconut milk gently, stirring occasionally to prevent scorching. Avoid bringing it to a boil.
- If you prefer a thicker consistency, add agar-agar powder to the coconut milk while it's heating. Whisk it in until fully dissolved. This step is optional and can be skipped if you prefer a thinner consistency.
- Once the coconut milk is warmed, remove it

from the heat and let it cool to approximately 110°F (43°C). You can use a food thermometer to monitor the temperature.

- Once the coconut milk has cooled, add the maple syrup or honey and vanilla extract. Stir well to incorporate the sweetener and flavoring.
- If using a yogurt starter culture, follow the package instructions to determine the appropriate amount to add. Alternatively, open the probiotic capsules and add the desired amount to the coconut milk. The amount can vary depending on the potency of the probiotic.
- Whisk the coconut milk and starter culture or probiotic together until well combined.
- Pour the mixture into clean glass jars or containers, leaving a bit of space at the top for expansion during fermentation.
- Cover the jars loosely with cheesecloth or a clean kitchen towel. This allows air circulation while keeping out contaminants.
- Place the jars in a warm spot, ideally between 105-115°F (40-46°C), to ferment. You can use a yogurt maker, an Instant Pot with the yogurt function, or simply place the jars in a warm oven with the light turned on.
- Allow the yogurt to ferment for 12 to 24 hours, depending on the desired tartness and thickness. The longer the fermentation, the tangier and thicker the yogurt will become.
- Once the desired fermentation time is reached, remove the jars from the warm spot and let them cool at room temperature.
- Transfer the cooled yogurt to the refrigerator and

let it chill for at least 4 hours or overnight. This helps it thicken further and enhances the flavor.

- Before serving, give the yogurt a gentle stir to incorporate any separated liquid and achieve a creamy consistency.

Sliced strawberries with coconut cream.

Ingredients:

- 1 cup sliced strawberries
- 1 can (13.5 oz) full-fat coconut milk, refrigerated overnight
- 2 tablespoons maple syrup or sweetener of your choice
- 1 teaspoon vanilla extract
- Optional toppings: shredded coconut, chopped nuts, or mint leaves

Instructions:

- Start by refrigerating the can of coconut milk overnight. This helps separate the thick coconut cream from the liquid.
- When ready to prepare the dessert, remove the can of coconut milk from the refrigerator without shaking or tilting it. Carefully open the can.
- You will notice that the thick coconut cream has solidified at the top of the can, while the liquid remains at the bottom. Scoop out the solid coconut cream and transfer it to a mixing bowl.
- Using a hand mixer or whisk, beat the coconut cream on medium speed for a couple of minutes

until it becomes smooth and creamy.

- Add the maple syrup or sweetener of your choice to the coconut cream. Also, add the vanilla extract for added flavor.
- Continue beating the coconut cream mixture for another minute or until the sweetener is well incorporated and the mixture has a fluffy texture.
- Wash and slice the strawberries. You can leave them as they are or gently mash a few slices to release some of the juices.
- In serving bowls or glasses, layer the sliced strawberries and spoonfuls of the coconut cream mixture. Repeat the layers until all the strawberries and coconut cream are used.
- Optional: Sprinkle shredded coconut, chopped nuts, or garnish with mint leaves on top for added texture and flavor.
- Serve immediately and enjoy the refreshing and creamy combination of sliced strawberries with coconut cream.

Baked cinnamon apples with coconut

Ingredients:

- 4 medium-sized apples (such as Granny Smith or Honeycrisp)
- 2 tablespoons maple syrup or honey
- 1 tablespoon lemon juice
- 1 teaspoon ground cinnamon
- 1/4 teaspoon ground nutmeg
- 1/4 cup unsweetened coconut flakes

Instructions:

- Preheat your oven to 375°F (190°C).
- Wash the apples thoroughly and pat them dry. Core the apples and remove the seeds, leaving the bottom intact to hold the filling.
- In a small bowl, combine the maple syrup or honey, lemon juice, ground cinnamon, and ground nutmeg. Stir well to create a smooth and fragrant mixture.
- Place the cored apples in a baking dish or on a baking sheet lined with parchment paper.
- Use a brush or spoon to generously coat each apple with the cinnamon syrup mixture, ensuring it fills the hollowed center and spreads over the skin.
- Sprinkle the unsweetened coconut flakes evenly over the coated apples, pressing them gently to adhere.
- Bake the apples in the preheated oven for about 25-30 minutes or until they are tender and the coconut flakes turn golden brown.
- Remove the baked apples from the oven and let them cool for a few minutes before serving.
- Serve the baked cinnamon apples warm as a delicious and healthy dessert. You can enjoy them as they are or pair them with a dollop of Greek yogurt or a scoop of vanilla ice cream for added indulgence.

Small piece of dark chocolate.

Ingredients:

- 1 small piece of high-quality dark chocolate (70% cocoa or higher)

Instructions:

- Start by selecting a high-quality dark chocolate that suits your taste preferences. Look for a dark chocolate bar with a cocoa percentage of 70% or higher, as this will have a richer and more intense flavor.
- Unwrap the dark chocolate bar and break off a small piece. The size of the piece can vary depending on your preference and portion control goals.
- Place the small piece of dark chocolate in a clean and dry dish or directly onto a serving plate.
- Enjoy the dark chocolate as it is, allowing it to slowly melt in your mouth, releasing its complex flavors and aromas. Take small bites and savor the experience.
- Optionally, you can pair the dark chocolate with a complementary ingredient like a small handful of nuts, a slice of orange, or a sip of black coffee to enhance the tasting experience.
- Remember to consume dark chocolate in moderation, as it is still a calorie-dense food. A small piece of dark chocolate can provide a satisfying and indulgent treat without excessive consumption.

Sliced mango with shredded coconut.

Ingredients:

- 1 ripe mango
- 2 tablespoons shredded coconut (unsweetened)
- Optional: a squeeze of lime juice or a sprinkle of chili powder for added flavor

Instructions:

- Start by selecting a ripe mango. Look for a mango that is slightly soft to the touch and has a fragrant aroma.
- Wash the mango and pat it dry. Using a sharp knife, carefully slice off both cheeks of the mango, avoiding the large pit in the center.
- Score the flesh of each mango cheek with a knife, making vertical and horizontal cuts to create a criss-cross pattern. Be careful not to cut through the skin.
- Hold the scored mango cheek and gently push the skin side up to invert the fruit. This will make it easier to remove the mango cubes.
- Using a spoon, carefully separate the mango cubes from the skin by sliding the spoon along the flesh, close to the skin. Repeat this process for the other mango cheek.
- Place the sliced mango cubes in a serving dish or bowl.
- Sprinkle the shredded coconut evenly over the sliced mango. You can use sweetened or unsweetened shredded coconut, depending on your preference for sweetness.
- Optional: Add a squeeze of lime juice over the mango slices for a tangy twist, or sprinkle a small amount of chili powder for a touch of heat and extra flavor.

- Gently toss the mango slices and shredded coconut together to coat the mango evenly and combine the flavors.
- Serve the sliced mango with shredded coconut immediately for a refreshing and tropical treat. Enjoy the juicy sweetness of the mango paired with the texture and subtle flavor of the coconut

Coconut milk-based ice cream.

Ingredients:

- 2 cans (13.5 oz each) full-fat coconut milk
- 1/2 cup sweetener of your choice (such as granulated sugar, maple syrup, or honey)
- 1 teaspoon vanilla extract
- Optional: add-ins such as chopped nuts, chocolate chips, or fruit

Instructions:

- Start by refrigerating the cans of coconut milk overnight. This will help separate the thick coconut cream from the liquid.
- Once chilled, carefully open the cans of coconut milk without shaking or tilting them. Scoop out the solid coconut cream that has separated at the top of the cans and transfer it to a mixing bowl. Discard or reserve the liquid portion for other recipes.
- Using an electric mixer or whisk, beat the coconut cream on medium speed until smooth and creamy. This step will help incorporate air into the

mixture and give the ice cream a lighter texture.

- Add the sweetener of your choice (such as granulated sugar, maple syrup, or honey) to the coconut cream. You can adjust the amount of sweetener based on your preference for sweetness.

- Add the vanilla extract to the mixture and continue to beat until all the ingredients are well combined.

- Optional: If desired, stir in any additional add-ins such as chopped nuts, chocolate chips, or fruit to enhance the flavor and texture of the ice cream.

- Once the mixture is ready, transfer it to an ice cream maker according to the manufacturer's instructions. Churn the mixture until it reaches a thick and creamy consistency.

- If you don't have an ice cream maker, you can pour the mixture into a shallow dish and place it in the freezer. Every 30 minutes, remove the dish from the freezer and vigorously stir the mixture to break up any ice crystals. Repeat this process several times until the ice cream becomes smooth and creamy.

- Once the desired consistency is achieved, transfer the ice cream to a lidded container and place it in the freezer to firm up for at least 2-4 hours or until it reaches the desired level of hardness.

- When ready to serve, scoop the coconut milk-based ice cream into bowls or cones. Garnish with your favorite toppings such as shredded coconut, chopped nuts, or chocolate sauce, if desired.

Baked cinnamon pears with honey

Ingredients:

4 ripe pears (such as Bartlett or Bosc)

2 tablespoons honey

1 teaspoon ground cinnamon

Optional: a sprinkle of nutmeg or a squeeze of lemon juice for added flavor

Instructions:

- Preheat your oven to 375°F (190°C).
- Wash the pears and pat them dry. Cut each pear in half lengthwise and remove the core and seeds using a spoon or melon baller. Place the pear halves in a baking dish, cut side up.
- Drizzle the honey evenly over the cut side of each pear half, allowing it to seep into the cavities. Use a spoon or pastry brush to ensure the honey coats the surface.
- Sprinkle the ground cinnamon (and nutmeg, if using) evenly over the pears, providing a fragrant and warming flavor.
- Optional: For a touch of acidity and to prevent browning, squeeze a little lemon juice over the pears.
- Place the baking dish in the preheated oven and bake for approximately 25-30 minutes, or until

the pears are tender and slightly caramelized.

- Remove the baked pears from the oven and let them cool for a few minutes before serving.
- Serve the baked cinnamon pears with a drizzle of the syrupy honey from the baking dish. You can enjoy them warm as a delightful dessert or as a topping for yogurt, oatmeal, or ice cream.

CONCLUSION

In conclusion, this book has explored the vital role that diet plays in managing interstitial cystitis (IC) and its impact on daily life. We have provided an in-depth understanding of IC, its causes, symptoms, and diagnosis, highlighting the complex nature of this condition.

Throughout the chapters, we have emphasized the significance of identifying and avoiding common triggers and irritants that can exacerbate IC symptoms. By adopting an IC-friendly diet, individuals can take control of their health and potentially alleviate the discomfort and pain associated with this condition.

We have discussed the impact of inflammation and how certain foods can either contribute to or reduce inflammation in the body. By choosing foods that are anti-inflammatory and nourishing, individuals with IC can support their overall well-being and potentially experience a reduction in symptoms.

The book has provided a comprehensive overview of

various food groups and their impact on IC symptoms, offering readers a valuable resource for making informed dietary choices. We have highlighted IC-friendly foods that are generally well-tolerated and can provide important nutrients while minimizing symptom triggers.

Furthermore, we have discussed the importance of personalized approaches to the IC diet, as each individual may have unique sensitivities and dietary requirements. Consulting with a healthcare professional or registered dietitian who specializes in IC can provide personalized guidance and support in creating a tailored diet plan.

By following the suggested meal plans, incorporating IC-friendly foods, and avoiding common triggers, individuals can optimize their nutritional intake while managing their IC symptoms. It is important to remember that dietary changes may take time and experimentation to find what works best for each individual, and patience is key in this process.

Ultimately, this book aims to empower individuals with IC to take control of their health and well-being through informed dietary choices. By adopting an IC-friendly diet and implementing the strategies outlined in this book, individuals can enhance their quality of life and find relief from the challenges posed by IC.

It is our hope that this book has served as a comprehensive guide, providing valuable insights, practical tips, and inspiration for individuals navigating the complexities of an interstitial cystitis diet. Remember, you have the ability to make a positive impact on your health and find a balance that works for you. Embrace the journey towards better health and know that there is support available every step of the way.